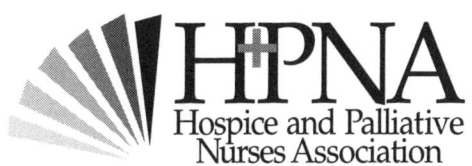

Compendium of Treatment of End Stage Non-Cancer Diagnoses

Dementia

Constance Dahlin, APRN, BC-PCM
Boston, Massachusetts

Patrick Coyne, MSN, APRN, BC-PCM, FAAN
Compendium Editor

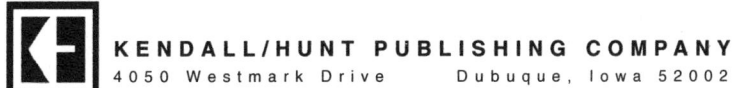

KENDALL/HUNT PUBLISHING COMPANY
4050 Westmark Drive   Dubuque, Iowa 52002

Copyright © 2006 by the Hospice and Palliative Nurses Association

ISBN 13: 978-0-7575-2546-9
ISBN 10: 0-7575-2546-6

Kendall/Hunt Publishing Company has the exclusive rights to reproduce this work, to prepare derivative works from this work, to publicly distribute this work, to publicly perform this work and to publicly display this work.

All rights reserved. No part of this publication may be reproduced, stored in a retrieval system, or transmitted, in any form or by any means, electronic, mechanical, photocopying, recording, or otherwise, without the prior written permission of the copyright owner.

Printed in the United States of America
10 9 8 7 6 5 4 3 2 1

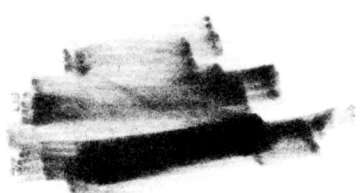

Contents

Expert Reviewers	iv
Disclaimer	v
Introduction	vii
Overview with Definitions	1
Types and Pathophysiology	2
Assessment	7
Early Interventions	10
Non-Drug Interventions in Late Dementia	13
Later Interventions	13
Psychosocial	20
Potential Research Issues/Opportunities	26
Cited References	28

Expert Reviewers

Judy Bartel, MSN, APRN, BC-PCM
Director of Clinical Programs
Hospice of the Western Reserve
Cleveland, OH

Frank D. Bellistri, MS, APRN, BC-GNP
Senior HEALTHWISE
Massachusetts General Hospital
Boston, MA

Patrick J. Coyne, MSN, APRN, BC-PCM, FAAN
Clinical Director of Thomas Palliative
  Care Services
Virginia Commonwealth University/
  Massey Cancer Center
Richmond, VA

Henry Farkas, MD, MPH
Medical Director
Seasons Hospice
Elkton, MD

Barbara Head, RN, CHPN®, ACSW
Research Director
University of Louisville, Program for
  Advanced Chronic Illness and
  End-of-Life Care
Louisville, KY

Judy Lentz, RN, MSN, NHA
Chief Executive Officer
Hospice and Palliative Nurses
  Association
Pittsburgh, PA

Maureen Lynch, MS, APRN, BC-PCM, AOCN
Nurse Practitioner
Dana Farber Cancer Institute
Boston, MA

Bridget J. Montana, MSN, APRN, MBA,
Chief Operating Officer
Hospice of the Western Reserve
Cleveland, OH

Dena Jean Sutermaster, RN, MSN, CHPN®
Director of Education/Research
Hospice and Palliative Nurses
  Association
Pittsburgh, PA

Disclaimer

HPNA will not be held liable or responsible for individual treatments, specific plans of care or patient and family outcomes. This compendium is intended for professional educational purposes only.

Introduction

As palliative care nursing continues to expand within the illness continuum and clearly beyond the population of oncology, nurses delivering this care must be knowledgeable in the current research and appropriate treatment strategies. This series of modules is designed to serve as a resource in constructing an appropriate plan of care for individuals and their families experiencing these diseases. These modules examine the incidence of each disease process, the pathophysiology of the illness, appropriate assessment techniques and treatments as the disease progresses. The modules further define the psychosocial implications. The modules specifically question the potential ethical, economic and research implication as related to each specific disease process. Each module was written by a nursing expert in the field and then reviewed by other expert clinicians of various disciplines to insure you the reader gain the best insight to helping your patients achieve the best quality of life possible.

Patrick J. Coyne, MSN, APRN, BC-PCM, FAAN
Clinical Director of Thomas Palliative Care Program
Virginia Commonwealth University/Massey Cancer Center
Richmond, VA

Overview with Definitions

Dementia results from a myriad of complex irreversible processes caused by changes in the brain that cause neuronal loss.[1] Due to the aging population, the number of people with dementia will increase at a dramatic rate in the next ten years. Some estimates are that in 2000, there were 4.5 million people with Alzheimer's disease. This will increase by 27 percent in the year 2020[2] and will result in a burgeoning strain on an already beleaguered healthcare system that is unprepared to care for these patients. This compendium section will emphasize the variety of dementia types and focus on palliative care for patients in the end stage of the disease.

The American Psychiatric Association[3] defines dementia as the development of deficits in memory, associated with deficits in one of the following areas: aphasia (language disturbances), apraxia (impaired ability to carry out motor activities despite intact motor function), agnosia (failure to recognize or identify objects despite intact sensory function) or disturbances in executive function (see Table 1). The World Health Organization[4] defines dementia as a sign of brain disease characterized by loss of mental powers. Dementia is characterized by intellectual deterioration while consciousness is maintained. Simply stated, dementia is the loss of mental functions. The disease continues to progress and the person regresses into almost a childlike being. The deterioration of the intellect causes degeneration of functional, motor, social and cognitive capacities. Specifically, memory loss, behavior, decision-making and language skills all irrevocably decline.[1]

Dementia is appropriately categorized as a progressive terminal illness. Volicer and Hurley[5] outline and describe four stages in the progression of dementia. In stage one, *mild dementia,* the patient experiences cognitive impairment. While still able to perform activities of daily living (ADLs), the patient is unable to perform more complex tasks such as cooking or shopping. In stage two, *moderate dementia,* the patient becomes more confused and apraxic, and unable to perform tasks. At this time, the patient may need help in activities of daily living with constant supervision at all times due to safety concerns. By stage three, *severe dementia,* the patient loses the ability for self-ambulation due to instability, and communication diminishes. Stage four, *terminal dementia,* marks the full decline and deterioration of the patient. The patient becomes bed-bound, uncommunicative and totally dependent in activities of daily living. He or she has difficulty eating or drinking and is highly susceptible to infections. Death, however, is not a direct result from dementia, but rather due to the many complications which occur during this vulnerable time.

TABLE 1 Dementia Criteria

I. Diagnosis made by impairment or decline in memory
II. Criteria
Aphasia–language disturbance or difficulty with any aspect of language Apraxia–inability to perform motor functions Agnosia–inability to recognize or identify objects Inability to perform executive functions such as planning, organizing, sequencing, abstracting

Reprinted with permission from the Diagnostic and Statistical Manual of Mental Disorders, Fourth Edition, Text Revision (© 2000). American Psychiatric Association.

There is a dearth of literature about end stage dementia in end-of-life literature. Since most of the research on end stage dementia has been done in Alzheimer's disease, it is well represented in the literature, while other forms of dementia receive little attention. The *Oxford Textbook of Palliative Nursing* devotes only two pages to dementia, and the *Oxford Textbook of Palliative Medicine* has only two paragraphs mentioning end stage dementia.

TYPES AND PATHOPHYSIOLOGY

In order to understand the pathophysiology of dementia, one must first understand the brain. The brain is a complex vital structure of the human body controlling all physical and cognitive functions. Weighing approximately 3-4 pounds, it is made up of an intricate network of blood vessels and some 100 billion neurons. There are three primary structures: the *brain stem,* responsible for basic survival activities such as breathing and heart rate; the *cerebellum,* responsible for balance and coordination; and the *cerebrum,* responsible for intellectual functions such as thinking, reasoning, analyzing, organizing, creating and decision-making.[6]

The cerebrum is divided into more discrete areas known as the left and right hemispheres, which are further divided into four lobes. The frontal lobe, located under the forehead, is responsible for personality. The parietal lobe, located behind the frontal lobe, receives sensory information and activates visuospatial movements. The temporal lobe, located near the temples, is responsible for hearing and language comprehension. The occipital lobe, located in the back of the head, is responsible for vision. Deeper within these structures are four important regions (the hypothalamus, the amygdala, the hippocampus, and the thalamus) that comprise the limbic system controlling emotions and motivation. The hypothalamus controls bodily functions such as eating, sleeping, sexual behavior, body temperature and hormone balances. The amygdala controls anger and fear. The hippocampus is vital for memory. The thalamus assists the brain in prioritizing information.[6]

The neurons within each of these structures allow communication to, from and within various parts of the body. The neuron structure includes a cell body with a nucleus, an extension called a dendrite that receives information from other neurons, and an axon that sends information to other neurons. Information is transmitted by neurotransmitters. These substances regulate and mediate chemical reactions within and between the neurons that produce electrical signals that initiate brain functioning. Proteins are essential to maintain the structure and function of neurons. In certain dementias, there is abnormal buildup of proteins within the neuron structure and alterations in levels of neurotransmitters resulting in malfunctions.[6]

At around age 50, the brain begins to shrink, most commonly in the frontal lobes. This atrophy is not as much as that which occurs in dementia. In dementia, the brain shrinks more extensively and may be marked in specific areas of the brain. These changes specific to each type of dementia can be detected using neuroimaging.[7] There are multiple causes of dementia ranging from Alzheimer's Disease, multiple strokes, infections in the brain, severe brain injury and thyroid deficiencies.[4] The specifics will be discussed under the description of the various dementias (see Tables 2 and 3). This section will discuss some of the more common progressive, irreversible causes that are seen in palliative care.

TABLE 2 Areas of Brain Affected by Dementia

Dementias–cortical and subcortical[8]

Cortical–outer layer of cerebrum that directs complex brain functions such as logic and reasoning. Tends to cause problems with memory, language, thinking and social behavior. Alzheimer's disease and frontotemporal dementia affect complex higher intellectual functions and produce early symptoms of planning and judgment[8]

Subcortical–affects areas of the brain below the cortex such as basal ganglia, thalamus, brain stem and motor coordination and vital functions. Tends to cause changes in emotions and movement in addition to problems with memory. Parkinson's and Huntington's chorea can cause movement disorders

Compiled from[8,9]

TABLE 3 Dementia Types

A. Reversible Causes

Cardiac disorders
Depression
Drug toxicity
Hydrocephalus
Brain lesions including hematomas and brain tumors
Metabolic disorders related to thyroid and parathyroid imbalances in sodium and sugar levels and liver function
Inflammatory diseases
Nutritional deficits–Thiamine (B1), Niacin (B6) and Folate (B12)

B. Irreversible Causes

Degenerative: Alzheimer's dementia, Lewy body disease, Pick's disease, Huntington's, amitrophic lateral sclerosis, Parkinson's
Vascular: multi-infarct disease
Cerebellar degenerations
Toxins: Alcoholism, heavy metals
Infections: Creutzfeldt-Jakob disease, HIV, neurosyphilis, tuberculosis, sarcoidosis
Neoplasms: primary or secondary tumors

Compiled from[8-10]

Alzheimer's Disease

Alzheimer's dementia (AD) is the most common type of dementia. It is the sixth leading cause of death for people 65 and over.[11] Currently, approximately 4.5 million have the disease. It is estimated to affect 3-5% of people over 65 with a prevalence of 23% in people who are 85 years and older.[12] With the prevalence doubling for each 5-year group after the age of 65, it is predicted that 13.2 million will be affected in 2050. Alzheimer's often goes undiagnosed in Hispanics and probably in other non-English speaking cultures, which makes further accurate estimates of incidence very difficult.[1] For these reasons, current incidence and prevalence are probably underreported and future predictions are underestimated.

Mitchell[11] found that 50% of nursing home residents were affected with Alzheimer's disease with individual care costs ranging from $42,000 - $72,000 a year. The course of disease is from 18 months to 27 years with an average range of 8-20 years and a median survival of 3-6 years.[1,10,11] It is characterized by memory loss, and behavioral changes such as social withdrawal and affective symptoms. This is accompanied by functional deterioration. Eventually, all of the areas are affected and the person is left with extreme deficits and total dependence on a caregiver.

Alzheimer's dementia was described in 1907 by Dr. Alois Alzheimer, who found abnormalities in the brain at autopsy of a patient who had died after lapsing into a progressive vegetative state.[10] Alzheimer's dementia is caused by the buildup of amyloid protein within the structure of neurons. Various hypotheses surrounding its etiology include: genetic predisposition indicated by family history, infection with a slow virus, aluminum toxicity, cholinergic effects of medications, autoimmune deficiencies, trauma and alterations in neurotransmitters.[6,10] Definitive diagnosis is achieved only by brain biopsy and evaluation for amyloid protein upon autopsy.[13]

The hallmark characteristics of Alzheimer's disease are the presence of neurofibrillary tangles (twisted protein fibers inside neurons) and neuritic plaques (protein between the neurons) as well as the loss of neurons in areas of memory and cognition.[1,13] Malfunctions of communication, metabolism and repair are evident in affected neurons. *Communication* relates to the integrity of neurons and appropriate synapses. *Metabolism* of the neuronal pathways is how molecules break down and generate energy. *Repair* refers to the maintenance of the neuron's structural integrity.

Plaques and tangles interfere with both the processes of communication and metabolism. The repair of injured neurons is impeded by the tangles, resulting in neurotransmission failure.[1] This causes subsequent alterations in the neurons, and further faulty neurotransmission that ultimately results in neuron death.[1] Several neurotransmitter imbalances appear to have a role in Alzheimer's disease, including acetycholine, dopamine, glutamate, norepinephrine and serotonin.[8]

The plaques and tangles are seen early in the hippocampus, which affect short-term memory. Changes can also be seen in the amygdala, progressing to the cerebral cortex where the functions of thinking and reasoning occur. When the cerebral cortex is affected, more severe cognitive changes occur along with sensory and motor deficits.[12] The overall effect is personality and behavior changes, deterioration in language and cognitive function, motor impairment and diminished self-care capacity.

Patients with Alzheimer's disease experience memory loss, as well as impaired ability to learn or retain new information and/or inability to attend to or focus on people or activities. Usually the first sign is loss of memory, which can be frightening to the patient.[10,14] Later, a patient's cognition, language, perception, praxis (the ability to order and coordinate movements and activities), problem solving, abstract thinking and judgment are affected. As the disease progresses, further changes develop in personality, cognition and social interaction. Functional changes occur in balance and gait. Neuromotor symptoms might include myoclonic jerks and generalized seizures, with accompanying oculomotor dysfunction.[10] Psychological symptoms include fearfulness, anxiety, paranoia and delusions accompanied by irritability, agitation and aggressive behaviors resulting in social withdrawal.

Vascular Dementia

Twenty percent of all dementias are of the vascular category.[9,15] This dementia is a cumulative clinical syndrome resulting from interruptions of blood flow to the brain from blockages or emboli. Vascular dementia (VD) may have an array of often overlapping causes, making it difficult to categorize and describe.[16] Some of the causes of vascular dementia include: 1] accumulation of small infarcts resulting from occlusion of branch arteries resulting in *lacunae* (small areas of fluid where brain matter used to be) and mental deterioration; 2] Binswanger's disease, which results in infarcts in subcortical white matter; 3] multi-emboli in any brain vessel; 4] vasculitis; 5] blood dyscrasias; 6] hypoperfusion often associated with vascular occlusion; and 7] anoxic episodes.[9,10,15]

Diagnosis may be complicated by the fact that a patient has both vascular dementia and Alzheimer's dementia.[6,14] The result is intellectual and functional impairment from cerebrovascular disease or continued cerebral injury.[8,10,16] There is research to suggest that a stroke may increase the later risk for dementia by nine-fold.[17] Other risk factors include old age, high cholesterol levels and high blood pressure. Clinical features include focal neurological signs and symptoms, depression, emotional lability, somatic complaints and nocturnal confusion.

Vascular dementia can occur insidiously or abruptly. In an insidious occurrence, only small areas are affected by vascular insufficiency or tiny infarcts from ischemia resulting in compromised cognition. As more vessels are blocked or develop infarcts, cognitive function further deteriorates. An abrupt occurrence may result from hemorrhage or anoxia, leading to severe and sudden cognitive decline.[10]

In the early stage, the patient may be afraid because they are aware of deficits, often resulting in depression. The patient may be emotionally labile and have somatic complaints. Nocturnal confusion can ensue. As vascular dementia progresses, there can be a sudden onset of deficits and/or stepwise decline in cognition, sensation and function.[12] In advanced states, a patient may become quite disabled and lose the capacity for continence, speech, ambulation, thereby becoming dependent in all activities of daily living. Treatment is limited and focuses on preventing further vascular disruption and preservation of function. This is achieved by maintaining normal blood pressure through the use of antihypertensive medications.

Lewy Body Dementia

Lewy body dementia (LBD) was first identified 40 years ago. According to the National Institute of Neurological Disorders and Strokes,[18] it is the second most common dementia. It is distinct from Alzheimer's dementia. Lewy bodies are abnormal egg shaped protein lumps composed of alpha-synuclein found in the cytoplasm outside brain nerve cell nuclei throughout the brain structure. They are present in 15-25% of patients who are autopsied.[18] These pathologic intracellular materials cause changes in the brain that result in cell death in the cortex of the brain and the substantia nigra of the midbrain.[18] They are found not only in the cerebral cortex or the brain stem, but also diffusely throughout the brain. LBD is highly associated with Parkinson's disease because the presence of such bodies in the brain stem is classified as Parkinson's disease.[12] The clinical presentation of Lewy body disease is similar to that of Alzheimer's dementia and Parkinson's disease with detailed visual hallucinations, delusions of persecution, impaired recent memory, muscle rigidity and fluctuating cognition. It may also have a more rapid progression than Alzheimer's.[19]

Frontotemporal Dementia

Frontotemporal dementia (FTD) is caused by degeneration of the brain, neuronal loss and gliosis of frontal and temporal lobes. This condition was first described in 1868 when Phineas Gage had a tamping iron bar impale his frontal lobe. The result was a changed personality where he became more disinhibited, raged in anger and frequently swore.[14]

Frontotemporal dementia is characterized by dysfunction in the frontal-subcortical areas that are necessary for self-monitoring, motivation and executive function. These patients typically have behavior, personality changes or problems with language expression.[14] Specifically, there is a buildup of tau protein within the neurons. Volicer et al.[16] describe the wide differences in classification of this condition within the mixed classification of dementias. Pick's disease is one variation of FTD. First described by Dr. Arnold Pick in 1892, it is characterized as frontotemporal lobar degeneration with argentophilic intranuclear inclusions or *Pick bodies*.[20]

Frontotemporal dementia is often overlooked or misdiagnosed, as it is difficult to distinguish from Alzheimer's. In the early stages, a patient may experience progressive language changes but, unlike AD, memory is initially spared. FTD symptoms include the development of loss of empathy towards others and lack of insight. With further progression, word-finding difficulties, compulsive eating, oral fixations and repetitive actions develop.[17] The final symptoms are loss of motor, speech and muscle weakness resulting in mutism, or the inability to talk or communicate. FTD usually develops in men and women from the ages of 35–70. There is a strong genetic predisposition.[17] Treatment focuses on managing residual effects of the dementia.

Alcohol-Related Dementia

Alcohol-related dementia is directly caused from alcohol abuse associated with a consumption rate of 150 ml of alcohol or more per day. This is the approximate equivalent of two bottles of wine, seven pints of beer or a half bottle of spirits. Chronic high alcohol intake has long-term metabolic effects related to deficiencies in thiamine, niacin and impaired liver function.[10]

If diagnosed early, this dementia is partially reversible with alcohol abstinence. However, in the case of chronic alcoholism, there is brain atrophy in the cortical and frontal areas. Liver damage causes increased ammonia levels that result in encephalopathy and neurological impairment. The clinical manifestations of encephalopathy are often mistaken for AD. However, alcohol-related dementia is milder because intelligence and language are spared.[8] Chronic thiamine deficiency, as seen in Wernicke-Korsakoff's disease, has irreversible effects on neuronal function in a small percentage of patients. Alcohol-induced pellagra (a niacin or tryptophan deficiency related to poor nutrition) causes brain lesions.[10]

Treatment focuses on alcohol cessation, vitamin supplementation and lactulose therapy to reduce and maintain lower blood ammonia levels.

HIV/AIDS Dementia

AIDS-related dementia, formally known as AIDS dementia complex, is caused by the HIV virus entering the brain cells. Usually it occurs after the development of several opportunistic infections that indicate severe immunosuppression. Before the introduction of the newer antiretrovirals, AIDS dementia was very common but it is now less pervasive with a prevalence of 7-27%. It is unclear if dementia rates will rise as HIV survival increases and there is greater longevity with advanced HIV infection.[21] AIDS dementia is considered a result of severe HIV-induced clinical manifestations in the brain.[21] HIV enters the central nervous system after initial exposure and causes pathological changes predominantly in the subcortical areas of the brain.[21] Specifically, the presence of the HIV virus promotes neurotoxins, such as cytokines and tumor necrosis factor, which damage neurons.[21] HIV dementia is broadly divided into two categories–a severe and a less severe form–which reflect the severity of the disease.

The virus manifests itself over time through a decline in cognition, motor function, and behavior change as damage occurs in the subcortical area of the brain. Progression is slow with subtle changes in neurological status. Cognitive changes include: impaired concentration and attention, impaired verbal memory, mental slowing, difficulty with calculations and abstractions, impairment of visuospatial memory, lack of visuomotor coordination and difficulty with complex task sequencing. In the late stages, decision-making, judgment and reasoning are affected.[8,22] Patients become confused, disoriented, aphasic and autistic. There is global cognitive impairment and mutism. Motor changes include behavior changes and gait disturbances.[22] The patient's behavior may be marked by psychosis, mania and inhibition. Delirium may occur secondary to the medications, acute infections or metabolic disturbances that cause hallucinations and delusions.[22] Fortunately, there has been a decreased incidence with newer antiretrovirals.

The actual diagnosis of HIV dementia is made by having an abnormal finding in at least two of the following areas: 1] attention/concentration 2] speed of processing or 3] abstraction/reasoning; and at least one of the following: 1] acquired abnormality in motor function, 2] performance, 3] decline in motivation or emotional control, 4] change in social behavior, 5] change in visuospatial skills, 6] change in memory learning, and 7] change in speech/language.[22] There are several risk factors for HIV dementia. These include: high plasma HIV RNA, low CD4 count, anemia, low body mass index, older age, intravenous drug use, abnormal constitutional symptoms prior to AIDS diagnosis and other co-morbidities.[22]

Unlike other dementias, HIV dementia can be determined with the assistance of several neuroradiologic studies. A magnetic resonance imaging (MRI) reveals diffuse enhancing white matter, cerebral atrophy and ventricular enlargement. A computerized tomography scan reveals brain atrophy, ventricular enlargement and increased white matter signal. Positron emission tomography and functional nuclear MRI reveal decreased metabolism in the thalamus and basal ganglia.[21]

End stage treatment focuses on continued antiretroviral therapy, including zidovudine and Tenofovir® (disoproxil fumarate), with the goal of preventing progression of cognitive decline and enhancing quality of life.

ASSESSMENT

History

Assessment of dementia begins with a medical review and history. The history should identify physical and behavioral changes that the patient and/or caregivers have noticed. A patient may not be a good historian because she/he has compromised recall and may not be able to articulate changes. Therefore, any information should be corroborated with the caregiver. The history should be collected with sensitivity to the patient's rights, privacy and in respect to their decision-making capacity. In end stage dementia, a history is best provided by family, friends and caregivers with close proximity to the patient, who may have clearly noticed changes. The focus remains on determining acute or insidious progression of mental impairments and changes in function, behavior or peculiar tendencies.

Pertinent questions to elicit information about changes in cognitive functions focus on memory and orientation, the patient's ability to perform activities of daily living as well as a review of emotional symptoms and behaviors.[10] Commonly described impairments include difficulty with familiar tasks such as food shopping, decline in job performance due to forgetting to do things, difficulty in language with inability to remember words or the name of objects, confusion of place and time with loss of sense of direction to places known to patients all their lives, lack of judgment demonstrated by performing odd actions at odd times, problems in abstract thinking evidenced by not being able to maintain money accounts, misplacing objects and putting them in strange places, mood fluctuations with extreme rapid outbursts, changes in personality with patients becoming the opposite of themselves and lack of initiative about simple tasks such as cleaning themselves or toileting. With this broad history, the pattern of cognitive deficits becomes clear. Safety becomes paramount to both the patients and their environment in terms of cleaning, cooking and other potentially harmful activities.

Physical Exam

For the initial diagnosis of dementia, a full neurological examination including evaluation of cranial nerve, motor and sensory function is warranted (see Table 4). Residual effects of stroke such as hemiparesis, hemisensory loss and visual field cuts may be confused with dementia, or indicate risk of vascular dementia. Loss of vibratory or joint position sense may be associated with alcoholism, nutritional deficiencies, infections and peripheral neuropathy. Extrapyramidal motor symptoms may include rigidity or slowness associated with Parkinson's, medication effects or dementia. Other symptoms of specific disorders include tremor, asterixis and gait abnormalities. The presence of primitive reflexes such as palmar grasp, palmomental reflex, snout reflex and glabellar tap are suggestive of dementia.

Evaluation of the patient's mental and cognitive status is often performed using the well-known Folstein Mini-Mental Status Examination (MMSE). This examination tests: orientation to date, time, and location; registration of three objects; attention and calculation; recall of the three objects; language in naming object, phrase and instructions; writ-

TABLE 4 Work Up for Dementia

CBC to rule out infection and anemia
Electrolytes panel to rule out glucose imbalances or calcium imbalances
BUN and creatinine to determine kidney function
Blood Ammonia Levels
Liver Function Tests to determine liver abnormalities
Renal Function Tests to determine kidney abnormalities
Thyroid Stimulating and Thyroid Function Test to determine abnormal thyroid levels
B12 for deficiencies
Folate for deficiencies
Heavy metal screening with history of exposure as appropriate
RPR for the presence of syphilis-induced dementia
Human Immunodeficiency Virus
Lyme disease
EKG for vascular dementia
Lumbar Puncture for meningitis/encephalitis, and measurement of amyloid and tau protein
Brain imaging for stroke
   Computerized Tomography
   Magnetic Resonance Imaging

C. Dahlin, 2006

ing a sentence; copying of two pentagons; and level of consciousness. While performing the exam, deficits in praxis (integration and performance of learned, complex motor acts) and visuospatial skills become evident. The MMSE may be used as a baseline for future testing to document declining function.[23]

Other laboratory work-up includes a full panel of blood and urine screening. This is to rule out signs of infections and other metabolic processes such as electrolyte abnormalities, hypothyroidism, B12 deficiency, renal disease and liver disease. Other neuroimaging such as brain imaging (computerized tomography, magnetic resonance imaging, positron emission tomography) and lumbar puncture may be warranted depending on the preferences of the patient and the family. Because there is no curative treatment of dementia, diagnostic testing is directed toward eliminating possible reversible causes and monitoring for co-morbidities.[8,10,24] In end stage dementia, workup revolves around clinical symptoms and reversible conditions. Treatment choices are made in accordance to the preferences, values and beliefs of the patient and family.

Functional Assessment

Ongoing assessment focuses on functional ability, safety and management of co-morbidities. As previously mentioned, Volicer and Hurley delineated the progression of dementia into four stages. The clinical dementia rating (CDR) evaluates memory, orientation, judgment and problem solving, community affairs, home and hobbies, and personal care.[25] CDR classifies severe dementia as the patient having severe memory loss, little or no orientation to people, inability to make judgments or problem solve, too ill to leave the house or care setting, no activities at home and requiring total care. Other tools used to document current functional status and track progressive changes in advanced dementia are the global deterioration scale (GDS) and the functional assessment staging test (FAST). These tools are useful in monitoring for declining function but are limited in projecting prognosis.[26] The GDS is a Likert scale from 1-7 that ranges from no cognitive decline to very severe cognitive decline. Reisberg and Ferris[26] describe severe cognitive decline at Level 7 as: all verbal abilities are lost, there may be no speech at all, patients are incontinent and need help with toileting and feeding, loss of basic psychomotor skills such as walking and the presence of generalized and cortical neurologic signs and symptoms.

The FAST tool assesses such tasks as normal functioning to difficulty remembering things, to difficulty traveling, inability to perform simple tasks, to the amount of assistance needed in personal care, to the ability to speak, smile, talk intelligibly and to hold one's head up. The range is from level 1 to level 7. Level 1 is no subjective or objective difficulty. Level 2 is forgetting location of objects and subjective work difficulties. Level 3 is decreased job functions and difficulty in traveling. Level 4 is decreased ability to perform simple tasks, finances, marketing or social gatherings. Level 5 is the necessity for help in dressing. Level 6 has five categories including patients' improper dressing, inability to bathe, inability to toilet and urinary and fecal incontinence. Level 7 has six categories including the patients' ability to speak only a few intelligible words, speech limited to one word and inability to ambulate, ability to sit up without assistance, to smile and hold up his/her head.[27] Patients in level 7 of both GDS and FAST scales are usually at the end stage of their disease and are appropriate for hospice. Luchins and Hanrahan[28] found that once patients were at level 7C of the FAST, the median life expectancy was three months. This meant the patient required assistance in ambulation, grooming, dressing, with the loss of continence and was unable to speak or communicate.

EARLY INTERVENTIONS

Alzheimer's Dementia

The two classes of medications most often used in the treatment of AD are cholinesterase inhibitors and glutamate inhibitors. Medications are used to slow progression or ameliorate symptoms.

Cholinesterase inhibitors stop or slow the action of acetylcholinesterase (an enzyme that breaks down acetycholine). This is important for the neurons located in the hippocampus that form memories. These medications can temporarily stabilize memory and reduce behavioral problems.[1,9,15] There are four drugs approved by the FDA:

- Donepezil (Aricept®)–restores level of function to that of 6-12 months before. Does not stop deterioration. Has relatively low side effect profile but can cause insomnia, agitation, leg cramps and GI upset. Dose is 5 mg/day increased to 10 mg/day after 4-6 weeks. Must be used cautiously in patients with peptic ulcer disease, asthma and bradycardia.[6,29,30]

- Rivastigmine (Exelon®)–similar to donepezil. Helps with memory. Initial dose is 1.5 mg BID, increased to 3 mg BID, to 4.5 mg BID to 6 mg BID with 2-week intervals between each dose escalation. Side effects include agitation and GI upset. Dose is 6-12 mg/day. Must be used cautiously in patients with peptic ulcer disease, asthma and bradycardia.[6,29,30]

- Galantamine (Reminyl®)–the newest medication. Improves cognition and behavior. Not as well studied. Side effects include GI upset. Dose is 16 or 24 mg day. Must be used cautiously in patients with peptic ulcer disease, asthma and bradycardia.[6,29,30]

- Tacrine (Cognex®)–dose QID with weekly escalations starting at 10 mg QID × 4 weeks, 20 mg QID × 4 weeks, 30 mg QID × 4 weeks, 40 mg QID × 4 weeks.[30]

Glutamate inhibitors are a newer drug class that act to regulate glutamate, a neurotransmitter that affects learning and memory.[9,15] There is only one glutamate inhibitor approved for use by the FDA:

- Memantine (Namenda®) regulates excess glutamate. Glutamate is involved in memory, but at high levels may cause damage to neurons.[1] Glutamate inhibitors work best in conjunction with cholinesterase inhibitors rather than alone.

Vascular Dementia

Treatment of vascular dementia includes management of high blood pressure to avoid further infarcts. Beta-blockers are recommended to maintain blood pressure within normal ranges. Anticoagulation therapy such as aspirin 81-325 mg day is also helpful. In addition, vitamin E 400-800 IU/day is thought to prevent further infarcts and to help maintain a healthy heart.[9,15]

Lewy Body Dementia

In Lewy body dementia, there tends to be less dopamine in the receptors resulting in parkinsonian symptoms. Logic would state that dopamine type medications, such as those used in treatment of Parkinson's disease, would be beneficial. However, such treatment in Lewy body disease may aggravate or worsen parkinsonian symptoms, rather than help them.[8,18] Neuroleptic medications may also worsen symptoms.[18] Selective serotonin reuptake inhibitors (SSRIs) can be utilized for depression. Beta-blockers are given for aggression, endocrine issues and hypersexuality. Benzodiazepines and typical antipsychotic agents should be avoided.[8]

Frontotemporal Dementia

In frontotemporal dementia, beta-blockers tend to help decrease and control aggression. Selective serotonin reuptake inhibitors (SSRIs) may help behavior problems. However, the patient should not be given benzodiazepines or antipsychotic medications because they can aggravate symptoms.

Alcohol-Related Dementia

Because long-term alcoholism tends to cause vitamin and nutritional deficiencies, the patient needs thiamine, niacin and nutritional supplements.

HIV/AIDS Dementia

The HIV dementia scale is more sensitive to subcortical psychomotor slowing in HIV than the mini-mental status exam. Antiretroviral medications should be continued to treat the HIV infection, and help maintain cognition. Medications include high doses of zidovudine (200 mg/day). Vitamin E and methylphenidate (Ritalin®) have also been shown to improve cognition and enhance functioning.[31]

Medications for Common Symptoms

There are many common symptoms in patients with dementia (see Table 5). These include behavioral and personality changes such as agitation and anxiety, delusions, hallucinations

TABLE 5 Clinical Features of Common Dementias

Features	AD	VD	LBD	FTD
Age of Onset	Usually after 65	Usually 60-75	Older adults	Usually 40-60
Pathology	Tangles and plaques	Infarcts	Cortical and brainstem Lewy bodies	Tau tangles
Affected Brain Areas	Hippocampus	Anywhere in brain	Substantia nigra of midbrain, cortex, cingulate gyrus, hippocampus	Frontal and temporal lobes
Cognitive Deficits and Clinical Features	Early memory loss Progressive decline Loss of orientation Personality and behavioral changes Memory impairment Hallucinations	Variable with site Stepwise progression Mood swings Stroke symptoms Depression Memory impairment Hallucinations	Variable Cognitive decline Hallucinations Parkinsonian symptoms Falls Memory	Personality and behavioral changes Lack of empathy Oral fixations Repetitive actions

Sources:[8,14,32]

and paranoia, psychiatric symptoms such as depression; and physical symptoms that include pain, incontinence, fever, insomnia. These symptoms may not appear in a systematic order, although they all present in the late stages of disease. Because of their side effect profile, it is difficult to predict which medication will be the most effective for a particular patient, making it essential to individualize management plans and to consider sequential trials of various medications in the class to find the most effective agent with fewest side effects.

Neuroleptic medications help manage aggression, agitation, restlessness, and are helpful for delusions, hallucinations and paranoia. Use of older anti-psychotics should be avoided due to the high side effect profile. Neuroleptic medications to manage symptoms including dopamine-blocking agents such as haloperidol, Risperdal®, olanzapine, clozapine.[24] Olanzapine has been found to be effective for vascular dementia.[33] Haldol® (2-3 mg/day) is effective but may bring on rigidity.[30] Clozapine (Clozaril®), risperidone (Risperdal®), quetiapine (Seroquel®) 0.5-10 mg/day and olanzapine (Zyprexa®) 2.5-5.0 mg/day may be alternatives with fewer side effects[6,34] (see Table 6).

There is some data on the use of beta-blockers to help agitation and aggression, perhaps by altering levels of norepinephrine. Suggestions are propranolol and pindolol 40-500 mg/day.[33] Additionally, some patients may have success with carbamazepine (Tegretol®) to help with agitation on doses of 400-1000 mg/day.[30]

Sleep disorders are also common. To help calm the patient and promote sleep, sedatives/antianxiety agents are helpful. However, caution should be utilized with benzodiazepines because they can worsen symptoms. To induce sleep, buspirone (BuSpar®), zolpidem (Ambien®) and trazodone (Desyrel®) are the best choices for medications as they affect serotonin levels.[24,34]

According to Volicer,[36] depression appears to be fairly common. The extent of this in late stage disease is unknown since patients lose the capacity to communicate such feelings. Depression may be difficult to distinguish from existential suffering. Antidepressants can readily treat depression. Therefore, a trial of serotonin selective reuptake inhibitors (SSRIs) is warranted. This includes Prozac®, Zoloft®, Paxil® or Celexa®.

AVOID DRUGS WITH ANTICHOLINERGIC ACTIVITY

The challenge of treatment according to Volicer[36] is that patients are unable to report side effects of treatment, and treatment interventions may be burdensome. Certain medications can be clearly problematic and should be avoided. DiTrapano[34] includes the following as medications to avoid since they can worsen symptoms and cause uncomfortable side effects: the antidepressant amitriptyline (Elavil®), the antipsychotic chlorpromazine (Thorazine®), the

TABLE 6 Symptoms of Dementia

Physiologic	Behavioral
Delusions	Aggression
Hallucinations	Agitation
Depressed mood	Wondering
Sleeplessness	Disinhibition
Anxiety	Screaming
	Swearing

Compiled from[35]

urinary spasmodic oxybutynin (Ditropan®), gastric antispasmodic hyoscyamine (Cystospaz®, Levsin®, also used to dry secretions) the antiemetics promethazine (Phenergan®) and prochlorperazine (Compazine®), the antihistamine diphenhydramine (Benadryl®) and two anti-Parkinson medications, trihexyphenidyl (Artane®) and benzatropine mesylate (Cogentin®).

OTHER MEDICAL INTERVENTIONS

Several medications have been studied with the hope of slowing progression of dementia. There have been various discussions of the use of vitamin E and selegiline. The American Academy of Neurology is clear that these agents should not be combined. Additionally, there have been suggestions that non steroidal anti-inflammatory drugs (NSAIDs) may slow progression of AD, but the evidence does not support this.[30]

Vitamin E is an antioxidant which may protect the brain from oxidation and which may retard progression of dementia.[1] Dosage is 1000 IU orally twice each day. Since vitamin E is an antagonist of vitamin K, it must be used with caution due to risk of bleeding in elderly patients who already may be on blood thinning agents.

In Europe, many patients with dementia are placed on ginkgo biloba. The range is 120-240 mg/day with the intent of protecting neurons from the oxidative damage from ischemia. Ginkgo biloba has been associated with increased risk of bleeding.[30]

NON-DRUG INTERVENTIONS IN LATE DEMENTIA

Memory Loss

Memory loss can progress rapidly. In earlier dementia, mental exercise to stimulate the brain may increase resistance to brain injury, stimulate new neuron formation and enhance cognitive and behavioral performance.[1] Reminiscence therapy and multisensory stimulation is also helpful to engage the cognitive aspect of the brain. In later stages, it is important to continue to engage the patient in mental exercise as much as possible as this helps behavior, decreases boredom and perhaps reduces depression. Often long-term memory remains intact; therefore, rote activities can be soothing and stimulating. Such activities can include folding laundry or towels, stacking things or squeezing a ball. Healing touch and massage can help with agitation. Physical exercise can decrease agitation and repetitive movements.

LATER INTERVENTIONS

Behavioral Changes

End stage dementias are associated with poor prognosis (see Tables 7, 8 and 9). There are many complications that arise with the continued progression of severe functional impairment and loss of cognition. Volicer et al.[37] created a nursing severity scale that examined dressing, sleeping, speech, eating, mobility, muscle strength and eye contact. The more dependent, disrupted, socially withdrawn, and weak the patient was, the closer the patient was to dying.

Both receptive and expressive aphasia with accompanying hallucinations result in increasing social withdrawal.[13,42] The physical changes that occur promote further confinement. The body can slow from rigid muscles. If the ability to walk is still present, there are severe gait disturbances.[42] Fall risk increases because of muscle weakness, poor coordination, failing judgment and forgetfulness. Decreased activity may predispose the risk

TABLE 7 Pain and Symptom Assessment

Change in vital signs	Facial expressions
Rectal exam	Slight frown
Urine dipstick and culture	Sad
	Frightened
Verbalizations/vocalizations	Grimacing
Sighing	Wrinkled forehead
Moaning	Closed or tightened eyes
Groaning	Distorted expression
Grunting	Rapid blinking
Calling out	
Noisy breathing	Body movements
Asking for help	Rigidity
Verbally abusive	Tenseness
	Increased rocking
Changes in interpersonal interactions	Restricted movement
Aggressive	Mobility changes
Combative	
Resisting care	Changes in activity pattern or routines
Decreased social interactions	Refusing food
Socially inappropriate	Change in appetite
Disruptive	Increase in rest or sleep periods
Withdrawn	Sudden cessation of common routines
Mental status changes	
Increased confusion	
Irritability or distress	
Crying or tears	

Compiled from[38,39]

of bedsores, thromboemboli and infections. Being immobile can also lead to incontinence, constipation and contractures. Sensory deficits may promote further frustration manifested in aggression and anxiety. Finally, cognitive decline may cause a failure to respond to or be aware of hunger. The patient seems to regress backward in time and in development towards an almost childlike personality. This, along with poor recall, attention and dysphagia, make the simple task of eating or feeding a prolonged event. Without attentive patient efforts on the part of caregivers, malnutrition and poor oral hygiene may occur.[43]

Additionally, there may be behavior issues such as sun-downing (late afternoon onset of agitation and confusion), which can be further exacerbated by alterations in sleep cycles.[42] These patients become very sensitive to and reactive to external stimuli.[42] Therefore, they need a calm and quiet environment without extraneous sounds, or sights such as television, radio or background noise. Daily routine helps soothe the patient. A well-lit room prevents delusions from shadows. Adhering to appropriate sleep cycles is important and decreasing afternoon naptime may promote sleep. A trial of sleep medications can be used once organic causes have been ruled out.

With progressive loss of cognition, emotion and motion, the patient's world dwindles, until they are essentially restricted and isolated in bed. There is the loss of meaningful interaction with the world and the inability to perform any self-care. These patients are prone

TABLE 8 Medications

Drug	Dosage Range
SSRIs for Depression and Agitation	
Sertraline (Zoloft®)	25-150 mg/day
Paroxetine (Paxil®)	10-50 mg/day
Fluoxetine (Prozac®)	5-20 mg/day
Citalopram (Celexa®)	20-60 mg/day
Venlafaxine (Effexor®)	50-300 mg/day
Sedatives for Sleep Disturbances	
Trazodone (Desyrel®)	25-50 mg/day
Zolpidem (Ambien®)	5-10 mg/day
Antipsychotics for Delusions, Hallucinations, Aggression	
Haloperidol (Haldol®)	0.25-5 mg Q 6 hours
Clozapine (Clozaril®)	75-100 mg/day
Risperidone (Risperdal®)	0.5-6 mg/day
Olanzapine (Zyprexa®)	2.5-20 mg/day
Quetiapine (Seroquel®)	100-250 mg/day
Agitation/Aggression Agents	
Buspirone (BuSpar®)	5-15 mg BID-TID
Carbamazepine (Tegretol®)	0-100 mg BID
Valproate (Depakote®)	125-250 mg/day

Compiled from[10,20,35,37]

TABLE 9 General Late Stage Dementia Characteristics

Onset–Insidious, chronic
Course–Long, no fluctuations during the day
Progression–Slow, may be fast at times and then plateau
Duration–Months to years
Awareness–Reduced or impaired
Alertness–Generally normal, but may become less alert
Attention–Generally normal but then become impaired
Orientation–Gradual impairment with severe impairment in late stage
Memory–Both short and long-term impairment at end stage
Thinking–Difficulty with abstraction and word finding, apraxia
Perception–Usually absent, may have misperceptions and hallucinations
Psychomotor Behavior–Apraxia
Sleep/Wake Cycle–Fragmented and altered
Affect–Variable
Family History–Potential in Alzheimer's, not in other dementia
Language–Limited vocabulary, severely impaired communication
Speech/Language–Dysphagia
Neurological–Gait disturbances, primitive reflexes, bowel/bladder incontinence
May vary by dementia type

Compiled from[12,40,41]

to skin breakdown and muscle contracture that may be painful. There can also be seizures or the development of paratonia (the involuntary resistance of arm or leg movement by another person). This reflexive process may be misinterpreted as aggressive behavior.

As the patient with dementia moves closer to death, he/she may be even more lethargic, and may develop cardiovascular and respiratory changes commonly seen in dying patients. Here the focus of care becomes energy conservation and comfort. The patient should receive assistance with all activities of daily living, meticulous skin care, soft covers to maintain warmth, and cool air to help breathing.[44] As with any terminally ill patient, respiratory distress may be treated with opioids.

Pain

Pain is often present in patients with dementia. All too often, patients with end stage dementia may be treated with antipsychotics and/or chemical and mechanical restraints for what may, in fact, be pain-related behavior.[11] One study found that nursing home assistants clearly identified loud/noisy behavior as pain behaviors.[45] Quieter patients were interpreted as depressed. So more education is needed for patients with dementia in long-term care settings.

Because patients may be restricted to a bed or chair, they may be predisposed to joint fatigue and bedsores. There may be co-morbid conditions such as arthritis, osteoporosis, cancer, peripheral vascular disease or diabetes that are painful. Bone tenderness and pressure may cause pain. The inability to communicate and report sensations makes pain difficult to assess. Pain is, therefore, probably greatly underreported and undertreated. Moreover, there may be the belief that pain is a function of aging.[46] There may be caregiver fear of pain medications and their potential side effects. Various studies further describe how patients with dementia thought to be in pain received less analgesia.[42,47]

Pain assessment can occur with both verbal and nonverbal patients. There are assessment scales for pain that ask patients to rate their pain from 1-10 or no pain to worse pain possible which can be difficult for patients with dementia who may not be able to perform abstract judgments. However, when asked about their pain, patients with dementia who are able to talk may attempt to describe pain in a more focused fashion. He or she may describe a sensation that may be more like a delusion such as being "shot" or "poked." Thus, the clinician should indeed assess the area in which he or she states to have been "shot" or "poked."

For non-verbal patients, pain assessment is measured through various behavior scales. The underlying theory is that pain manifests itself as change in activity, vocalizations, delusions, hallucinations, combativeness, pulling away when touched, splinting a body part, or withdrawal.[12,36,42] There also may be changes in behavior. For instance, a patient who is outgoing may become withdrawn and a patient who is quiet may become noisy and loud.

The American Geriatric Society Panel (AGS) on Persistent Pain in Older Persons[39] suggests evaluating the following areas: facial expression, verbalizations, body movements as well as changes in interactions, in routines and mental status. Facial expressions include a frown, sad face, frightened face, grimacing, wrinkled forehead, closed or tightened eyes or some type of distorted expression. Verbalizations include moaning, groaning, sighing, grunting, calling out, noisy breathing, asking for help or verbally abusive behaviors. Body movements include rigidity, guarding, fidgeting, pacing, rocking, restricted movements and mobility changes. Changes in interpersonal interaction include aggression, combativeness, withdrawal or socially inappropriate behavior. Changes in routines include refusal of food, changes in appetite, increase of rest periods, changes in sleep patterns or changes in common routines. Mental status changes include increased irritability, confusion or distress.

There are several helpful scales for patients with dementia. All assess the various areas as suggested by the AGS although some focus solely on facial expressions, verbalizations and body movements. Among them are the Abbey pain scale, Assessment of Discomfort in Dementia (ADD) protocol, the Checklist of Nonverbal Pain Indicators (CNPI), the Discomfort Scale –Dementia of Alzheimer's Type (DS-DAT) and Pain Assessment in Advanced Dementia scale (PAINAD).[48-51]

To assess pain, it is recommended that clinicians use the PAINAD scale. This is a five-item scale that combines elements of the discomfort scale for patients with dementia of Alzheimer's type (DS-DAT) and a pain scale for dementia developed previously by Volicer and his colleagues.[51] The scale evaluates the presence of noisy breathing, negative vocalizations, facial expressions, body language and consolability.[52]

Once pain is suspected, it important to identify the etiology which may be extremely difficult in the non-verbal patient. If pain is suspected, a trial of analgesics can be instituted. If the result is that the patient seems calmer, more relaxed and less agitated, the pain medicine becomes the diagnostic indicator and the pain diagnosis is established.[12] As for all geriatric patients, the rule is to start low and titrate up slowly, reassessing frequently. Clinicians should tailor therapy to disease specific types of pain making use of acetaminophen, nonsteroidal anti-inflammatory drugs, local anesthetics and opioids. Sometimes just 1 mg of morphine or 0.5 mg of hydromorphone can help these patients by treating chronic pain. If these patients are hospitalized, pain history and assessment should occur and therapy initiated per American Pain Society and American Geriatric Society Guidelines.[39]

Depression

Patients with dementia may also experience depression. However, it is difficult to assess since these patients are non-verbal and unable to express their thoughts and feelings. Instead, depression may manifest itself in changes of behavior, with the patient becoming more withdrawn or refusing food. This may happen when there is a change in environment.

Patients with dementia respond to antidepressant medications. Therefore, it is worth a trial of medications if pain has been ruled out.[53] The result may be that the patient is more attentive and has interest in food.

Constipation

It is paramount to document bowel activity with early interventions for altered bowel patterns to avoid unnecessary and painful impactions. Compromised ability to eat and limitations in activity, as well as use of certain medications, predispose patients with dementia to constipation. Moreover, if a pain regimen is initiated, an accompanying bowel regimen should be instituted. Constipation can exacerbate urinary incontinence and increase risk of infection. Therefore, an appropriate bowel regimen should be initiated. Because many of these patients cannot eat or drink adequately, bulk-forming laxatives and stool softeners alone are ineffective. Instead, mild laxatives including oral senna with docusate are the mainstay of therapy. If ineffective, the routine use of a stimulant laxative suppository or an enema may be necessary.[44]

Skin Integrity

Compromise in skin integrity can result from poor self-care. Later in the disease, apraxia, dysphagia, decreased mobility and incontinence increase the risk for decubitus ulcer formation.[42]

Nutritional supplements can enhance protein levels to maintain the skin. Routine inspection of the skin can lead to early intervention. Efforts to reduce sustained pressure include frequent position changes, special mattresses and chair pads and other pressure-reducing devices. Sometimes home care or hospice nurses may use DuoDERM® or Tegaderm® to protect pressure areas from breakdown. Patients with dementia need to be encouraged or assisted to change positions in a calm, gentle fashion. These patients have fragile skin and are at risk for shearing and tears just from being moved. The use of assistive devices is strongly encouraged. Bathing is very important to remove soil, urine and fecal material. However, care and consideration should be given to the method. In end stage, patients cannot tolerate showers or baths as these cause anxiety, fear and increased agitation. Bag baths are recommended at this stage.[54]

Pain and infection are complications of bedsores. However, topical opioids may be a potentially helpful intervention rather than oral opioids that may cause more sedation. After cleaning the ulcer site, a concentration of morphine 0.1mg per 1 unit solution may be added to a dressing gel and applied one to two times a day.[55]

Incontinence

Since patients lose bladder and bowel continence, protocols for routine toileting and cleansing of the perineal area need to be established and followed as per the Agency for Health Care Policy and Research Guidelines.[56] The American Academy of Neurology supports behavior modification, scheduled toileting and prompted voiding to reduce urinary incontinence.[30] When the patient is bedridden, the use of absorbent pads and barrier products can help protect the skin. These measures also help avoid the frequent potential of urinary tract infections if patients are left sitting in urine or stool.

Infections

Changes in the immune systems, less activity, incontinence and dysphagia are contributing factors for high infection rate in patients with dementia. In particular, patients with dementia have a high rate of pneumonia, urinary infections and decubitus ulcers. Additionally, this older cohort may have other common co-morbidities such as coronary artery disease, hypertension and congestive heart failure, which complicate care.

Pneumonia, with recurrence, is a particularly common issue as patients become too weak to swallow effectively and aspirate.[57] Volicer,[36] Mitchell,[11] and Morrison and Sui[58] all found that at least 50% of patients with end-stage dementia die from pneumonia. The quandary is how to best treat pneumonia while considering the benefits and burdens of care with the goal of maintaining comfort. The standard of care includes radiographic studies, blood work and insertion of a line to deliver intravenous antibiotics. These measures usually necessitate a hospital admission.

The work-up can be overwhelming to these patients and can cause more distress than the infection itself. In particular, blood drawing is more upsetting to the patient due to lack of understanding about its necessity and inability to comprehend the reason for the pain.[36] Radiographic testing may be too confining and overwhelming. Treatment can also be controversial since there is no consensus of standard therapy. Van der Steen et al.[59] found that treatment with antibiotics may reduce discomfort. Nonetheless, issues of oral versus intravenous antibiotics, the role of intravenous fluid replacement, the use of oxygen therapy or more aggressive respiratory support, and hospitalization should be resolved in the context of the patient's overall condition and goals of care.[47]

Volicer[36] suggests antibiotic therapy for the first isolated episode of pneumonia. Oral antibiotics are better tolerated with fewer side effects including gastrointestinal upset, diarrhea and allergic reactions. Aggressive treatment of infections does not necessarily prolong survival and may accelerate severity of disease.[47] Pinderhughes and Morrison[57] suggest that if the patient becomes febrile, treatment should be palliative and should be solely focused on symptomatic relief and eliminating discomfort. These measures include the use of antipyretics, management of secretions for comfort, opioids for dyspnea and the exclusion of extraordinary measures.

Urinary tract infections are also common. Asymptomatic bacteruria may not require treatment but it is important to remember that in many patients with dementia the typical symptoms of dysuria, urgency and frequency are absent. Changes in behavior such as increased aggression, agitation, malaise may be more sensitive indicators of infection. Incontinence, urinary catheters and poor fluid intake may predispose the patient to infection. Obtaining urine specimens, especially clean specimens, can be difficult and the trauma of catheterization needs to be carefully considered in light of treatment goals. Issues in treatment are similar to those with pneumonias.

Nutrition

Functional and cognitive decline necessitate diet modifications, individually tailored meal plans and feeding schedules. The availability of finger foods may tempt some patients to self-feed but in advanced stages, hand feeding may be necessary. Foods with strong or sweet flavorings may be preferred since patients with dementia may lose the ability to taste. If patients prefer sweets, protein enrichment helps decrease the intake of empty calories.[43]

Malnutrition often occurs because patients lose interest in food, forget how to swallow, lose the ability to swallow effectively and experience decreased appetite. It becomes a vicious cycle, since as appetite declines, malnutrition and dehydration may ensue. Malnutrition and dehydration in turn promote further decline. Moreover, patients may no longer recognize food, or accept it into their mouth. If the patient does readily accept food, the process of feeding may be burdensome and cumbersome for the caregivers. The need for longer feeding times may test a caregiver's patience and energy. As eating times become more prolonged, considerations of benefits and burden of feeding may become a topic of conversation.

Dysphagia

In terminal dementia, dysphagia is common due to decreased consciousness from the disease itself or as a side effect from various medications needed to manage behavior issues.[40] To promote maximal safe swallowing, feeding should take place in a relaxed quiet atmosphere. The patient should be positioned upright appropriately in a chair or bed with the head elevated to avoid a compromised airway and gastroesophageal reflux.[40] The patient may need stimulation and cueing with feeding utensils.[43,40] In the very end stages, patients may be able to take very small sips of thicker substances.[40] Smith[44] suggests that the patient be offered cool, not cold, thick drinks such as melted ice cream, smooth fruit or yogurts.

Tube Feeding

Tube feeding is a controversial topic. Palliative care and gerontologists agree that the burdens of care often outweigh the benefits of care. Research on care in nursing homes demonstrates there is a tendency of nursing home administrators to encourage tube feedings in spite of the problems associated with inserting feeding tubes.[11,60-62] In fact, 30% of patients get tube feedings. Although feeding tubes may provide artificial nutrition and hydration, problems such as diarrhea, tube patency issues, skin infections and patients' requiring restraints to keep them from pulling tubes out may occur.[63] Additionally, there is the continued risk of aspiration.

Research studies have shown that feeding tubes in patients with dementia do not prolong survival nor do they promote quality of life.[11,60-63] Rather, it may be better to provide mouth care to prevent the discomfort of dry mouth rather than aggressive measures to maintain hydration. However, discussion about goals of care is paramount to allow families to understand the benefits and burden of such interventions. Families may be guided by considerations in the ethics literature, which state that feeding is not necessary if it is burdensome, and a Supreme Court decision that tube feedings constitute a medical treatment that may be properly refused by the patient or his or her healthcare proxy.[63]

Hospitalization

Although optimal care of end stage dementia does not include hospitalization or even admission to the intensive care unit, many patients do end up there. The number of admissions is expected to increase as the number of patients with dementia increases.[64] These patients are often hospitalized for urinary infections, pneumonias and decubitus ulcers. These admissions, however, are difficult for these patients. Patients with dementia are weak, with respiratory insufficiency and meet hospice level of care as they have a poor functional status. Additionally, the patient with dementia may experience pain from multiple causes including the care from the illness (such as phlebotomy), chest tubes, placement and removal of intravenous catheter, dressing changes, endotracheal tubes and/or suctioning. They may become agitated in the unknown surroundings with the many procedures and be slow to respond to therapy.

Often these hospitalizations occur because there is no indication of advance care planning discussions and full resuscitative measures are default until such discussions change the goals of care. To facilitate the redirection of care from curative to supportive, an ethics or palliative care consultation may be a helpful approach. Campbell and Guzman[64] suggest screening the medical intensive care unit for patients who are 80 or older with a diagnosis of dementia and decubitus ulcers or pneumonia. With permission from the team, the families or decision makers of these patients are then contacted for family meetings to discuss goals of care. With discussion, these patients can then more appropriately receive supportive care, either in the hospital or with a transfer to a hospice setting. The focus is then on pain for ulcers and distress and supportive measures for infections such as antipyretics and opioids for dyspnea.

PSYCHOSOCIAL

As the ability to independently participate in activities declines, the patient systematically loses functional ability and possibly his or her dignity. The patient needs assistance in performing the simplest of tasks, becoming more isolated from the world as s/he remains in their house, room or bed. This may lead to social isolation, anxiety and depression.

Non-pharmacological interventions to improve psychological engagement include presence of known caregivers and family, familiar and patient-preferred music, light exercise and assistance in movement as appropriate. Neutral colors, decreased noise and moderate temperatures are also helpful in creating a more relaxed environment.[35] Music therapy has been found to significantly improve speech and fluency for dementia patients.[65] Pet therapy has also been found to be helpful.[30] Additionally the continuation of familiar religious ceremonies, hymns and spiritual rituals help give some support and calming influence to patients with dementia.[66] Aromatherapy has also been found to be calming for these patients. In essence, minimizing challenges to lapses in memory and invoking pleasant sensations may ease episodes of anxiety, aggression or withdrawn behavior.

Safety

Safety is paramount and nonnegotiable.[8] Since patients have lost their judgment, they often do not understand the risk associated with their actions. Therefore, the family needs to manage safety beginning with the home. A safe home environment may mean the removal of toxic chemicals, sharp instruments, tools and stove knobs. Bright, but not harsh, lighting can help maintain orientation. Removal of clutter can help decrease confusion and minimize the risk of falls. Assistive devices such as safety rails on the bed and in the bathroom are necessary for both the patient and the family due to the potentially deleterious effects of a fall for the patient or caregiver. Removal of unnecessary locks (for example those on bathroom and bedroom doors) is necessary. Environmental modifications, behavioral interventions and non-sedating medications should be thoroughly exhausted before the use of physical restraints is considered. Physical restraints should be used cautiously and with consideration of the benefit and burden of such measures. They may cause more potential problems by increasing combative behavior, confusion and disorientation. It may be necessary to sedate the patient particularly if there is not twenty-four hour help.[16,36] If falls are an issue, mattresses can be placed on the floor.

Communication

Communication for patients with dementia is affected as the disease progresses and becomes more difficult. Continued verbal communication from caregivers is vital in helping these patients remain socially engaged. There are many suggestions for communicating with patients with dementia. Most important is the necessary patience and understanding by healthcare providers and caregivers as any interaction will take longer. All too often caregivers become fatigued by the demands of care, become frustrated and react negatively to these patients. They may argue with patients, order them around and infantilize them. This is demeaning and disrespectful, causing much distress for patients who may still understand the tone and non-verbal cues of such interactions.

To begin with, communication should occur in a calm atmosphere without radio or television distraction. Patients first need to be cued to the presence of another person in a calm manner. The caregiver should speak in a low pitch to promote the patient's ability to hear. Verbal expression should include the use of simple words and sentences, repetition of sentences, explanations of what is to happen and descriptions and demonstrations of what needs to be done. Slang or idioms should be avoided and the use of common courtesies should be continued. For these patients, only one question, direction or comment can be made at a time. If patients are given choices, they should be simple and positive.[12,43] Most successful are positive suggested actions such as "Let's do this," or "Shall we try this?" Otherwise, these patients get frustrated leading to further agitation and combativeness.

Non-verbal cues include moving slowly to the patient, maintenance of eye contact as well as provision of a comforting and patient touch. Smiling, nodding and the use of touch can help calm a patient. These patients are reassured with the continued presence of the person by their side. In the very end stage of dementia, patients may not be able to vocalize or verbalize anything intelligible. It is still necessary to cue patients and alert them to activities such as personal care and moving.

Social Interaction

Social isolation unfortunately occurs all too soon, frequently due to lack of communication and withdrawal from daily routines. Furthermore, in late stages, these patients are bed-bound and are often alone and isolated in bedrooms. Offering nursing presence and some small interaction in short periods of time can promote comfort, dignity and self worth. Moreover, these patients often need reassurance during all activities or interactions. Soothing and supportive verbal communication can be effective.[38] This includes talking to them while assisting with any personal care and being very sensitive to maintaining privacy while assisting with activities of daily living.

Head[43] offers two techniques: bridging and chaining. Bridging allows the patient to hold an item similar to that of the caregiver, which connects them to the activity as past memory may be stimulated. For instance, both may hold a handcloth for washing. Chaining is where a caregiver helps a patient through the initial parts of a task and then the patient may finish as memory of the activity is stimulated. For instance, the caregiver starts to button a shirt and then the patient continues.

Other soothing activities include the use of sensory objects and busy hand activities, music therapy including group sing-alongs, pet visits, listening to poetry and/or short stories based on the patient's preferences and personality.[67] When a person is bed-bound, supportive touch, massage and gentle physical movement or therapy can be helpful.[38]

Advance Care Planning

Advance Care Planning is optimally discussed before a patient develops any condition. Morrison and Sui[58] found that in their study of 118 patients with dementia, only 10% had such documentation of any discussion about goals of care. This includes the issue of medical futility if the disease is incurable. For these patients, the rate of successful resuscitation is low and treatment does not prolong life. Hospital transfer puts patients more at risk causing more falls and infections. Realistic decision-making early in the disease can help the patient receive appropriate care in the comfort of the setting the patient knows best. This avoids fear and unnecessary tests that will not change the outcome of the disease.

The importance of getting affairs in order in the earliest stages of the disease when memory and intellectual functions are intact cannot be emphasized enough. Designation of a healthcare agent determines who will make healthcare decisions when the patient is unable to make decisions. A *living* will is a document that outlines the type of care a patient would like to receive within certain medical situations. A *durable power of attorney* designates a person to make financial decisions for the patient when they lose decision-making capacity. A *will* is a document that divides assets after a person's death. Other business affairs pertain to finances around future care needs, exploring insurance coverage and organizing paperwork for caregivers.

Ideally, this should include short and long-term care issues such as help at home, day care, nursing home placement, specialty units and hospice. It is important to facilitate the discussions patients and families have regarding the use of aggressive life sustaining treatments, quality of life concerns and completion of the legal paperwork for a healthcare proxy or living will. Particular to this population, it is helpful for patients and families to have realistic information such as the low rate of successful CPR and the increased risk of infections and falls with transfers to the hospital.

Nurses can offer resources and information along with documentation in the medical record about such discussions. In promoting advance care planning, it is important that the nurse understands his/her state laws to guide the family. The Patient Self Determination Act of 1991 made it necessary for every state to have a document about healthcare proxies. However, these may not be recognized in other states. Furthermore, not every state recognizes living wills. Many states have out-of-hospital comfort care forms, while some have do-not-resuscitate orders recognized by emergency medical systems. When completed, all of these forms are helpful documentation to guide decisions. However, the most important act is having the conversation to discuss a patient's values, beliefs and preferences in life sustaining therapies and their definition of quality of life.

Family

FINANCES

It is estimated that caring for persons with dementia costs at least 100 billion nationally or $47,000 per person per year.[1,8] This cost may reflect only the healthcare costs, but there are also personal costs incurred by families who care for persons with dementia. Most patients with dementia are cared for in the home.[68] When extra care is needed, many families pay for this privately. Nursing home care is not usually covered under state aid, as it is custodial care. Providing custodial care within the family often means lost employment and a threat to financial security. Additional costs of care include hired respite caregivers or nursing home stay, uncovered medication costs, protective devices, incontinence pads, nutritional supplements, and transportation, all of which can be expensive, particularly with the changes in Medicare coverage.

HOME CARE SUPPORTS

More recent work by Mitchell et al.[11] found that only 1- 4% of patients in home hospices had a dementia diagnosis while 7-16% for patients in long-term facilities carry a dementia diagnosis. Patients cared for at home are less demented, less debilitated, have fewer behavior problems, and require fewer feeding tubes than those in an institution.[11,53] Many patients do not receive home care since dementia is a long-term chronic illness in which the patients do not fit the home health/homebound criteria until very late stage.

The NHO Medical Guidelines of 1996[69] states a patient should need 'total care'. This includes inability to independently perform the following: ambulation, dressing, properly bathing, toileting, controlling bowel and bladder, speaking or communicating meaningfully or maintaining sufficient calories or fluids compatible with sustaining life. Moreover, they should have co-morbid conditions such as aspiration pneumonia or an urinary tract infection, septicemia, multiple stage 3-4 decubitus ulcers and recurrent fevers. Sachs[42] offers other critical times for hospice consideration. They are: 1] the combination of loss of meaningful communication, weight loss of 10% or more, recurrent infections, and multiple pressure sores, 2] hip fracture or pneumonia and 3] need for a feeding tube to maintain nutritional status. The hospice may be able to offer support to family caregivers with the use of volunteers, allowing for time out and ventilation of thoughts and feelings. When patients do not meet hospice criteria, palliative care programs may offer much needed supportive care and ongoing caregiver information.

However, this criteria has been found to be inadequate as a prognostic tool for dementia because dementia is unpredictable.[70,71] Only 7% of hospice patients have a diagnosis of dementia.[72] Around 10-15% of patients have a secondary diagnosis of dementia and it is expected that those numbers will rise.[73]

This means the majority of care is given by caregivers and many families do not have a support network or care coordination.[74] This promotes further stress and caregiver fatigue. When these patients are in hospice, they enroll for a median of several months.[70,73]

Adult day care centers may be an option for some families. These full and half-day programs can be located in the community or associated with a medical center. Usually, there is structured time and lunch is provided. Personal care and medical attention may be offered. These services can offer some respite to the family from the constancy of caregiving. They can also offer a supportive environment to help ease the emotional burdens of the care. These programs are less expensive than a skilled nursing facility. However, they may still be a financial burden for some families. Moreover, they may not be available in many communities and some may not have the expertise to handle these patients.

Respite care is another possibility. Sometimes other family members or members of a religious or spiritual community can provide intermittent respite. However, caregivers need more prolonged breaks. With this focus, a patient is admitted to an extended care facility for a couple of days to allow the family to rest. This may occur under private pay instances, in collaboration with an Alzheimer's Association, or under hospice.

Finally, there are long-term care facilities. Many patients with dementia will be in nursing homes for about 25% of their care.[75] Families looking for facilities will find dramatic differences in quality.[20] Few are devoted exclusively to the care of demented patients. Some may have a dedicated unit or a mix with general geriatric population. The considerations for nursing home choice are based on cost, proximity, physical environment, cleanliness, staffing, familiarity of caring for dementia patients, quality of care and programs.

Another very important consideration with end stage dementia is the care philosophy. For some facilities, there is conflict between nursing home regulatory guidelines and the palliative care focus for end stage patients with dementia.[62] Johnson[62] discusses how the physical signs that are common to the dying process are interpreted as failures on the part of the nursing home. This inhibits good palliative care and may explain the high rate of imminently dying nursing home patients who are transferred to the hospital.

Hurley and Volicer[53] offer several criteria to consider when selecting a nursing home. First, there is the safety of the physical environment, including whether or not a unit is locked, the precautions to prevent escape, fall prevention, the use of physical and chemical restraints and the use of assistive devices. Second, there is the dementia-specific health management provided to the patient. This includes the frequency of routine healthcare visits by a physician or nurse practitioner, the use of memory-enhancing medication and the use of cognitive-enhancing activities. Third, there is the overall attention to the health of the patient. Under this category is the breadth and depth of medications and treatments that can be managed without hospital transfers, the assessment and management of chronic and new health problems, the protocol for determining the need for acute care, and the availability of hospice and palliative care services. Fourth, there is the knowledge and availability of staff, particularly as the dementia becomes end stage. This category includes the type and frequency of staff education, the percentage of nursing assistants and nurses who are certified in geriatric or hospice and palliative care of dementia patients, the availability of special consultants and the patient-to-registered nurse ratio. Fifth, there is the attention to quality-of-life issues, including programs to maintain optimal physical functioning, the existence of a pain management program, and ongoing activities. Sixth, there is the presence of support groups for family as well as family education programs. Finally, the last issue pertains to the use of an interdisciplinary team, the frequency of each member's evaluation, and use of family meetings. Considering each of these areas can help a family member find a nursing home that focuses on attentive palliative care for end stage dementia patients. It may also promote a placement that relieves that family of the guilt and burden of needing to put a patient in a skilled facility when there is a good philosophical fit for end stage dementia care.

CAREGIVER FATIGUE

Caregiver fatigue is unending as patients with dementia need constant supervision due to safety and weakness. Their care is also draining because of the patient's behavioral issues and emotional lability. If patients are experiencing altered sleep cycles, there is never time to rest. Sleep deprivation can be debilitating without opportunity for rejuvenation. It can also lead to mental and physical illness for the caregivers. Many families cannot afford to pay for extra help so depend on other family members and friends for even short respites. There is growing evidence that the amount of annual expenditures for dementia care includes the health toll on caregivers.[2]

Often caregivers of dementia patients need respite or rest away from caregiving. These caregivers may find some respite available through Elder service programs, Alzheimer's Organizations and with volunteers through hospice. Often, they must rest while home health agency nursing assistants are present. Some may find family, friends, church or community members who are willing to provide some discrete hours of help. Other times, caregivers must utilize appropriate sleep medications to get rest at night. However, this may not be enough and the caregiver may need an extended break from care such as days to weeks. The chronic fatigue is a factor in the placement of many patients with dementia into long-term care facilities.

CAREGIVER COPING

The emotional impact of caring for patients with dementia can be all consuming and overwhelming. The constant necessity of care translates into little personal time or breaks from caring. Moreover, the toil of the sacrifice goes unappreciated and unnoticed by the patients with dementia. To cope with the range of emotions, caregivers need contact with professionals such as nurses, social workers, psychologists, pastoral care and support groups.[2,76]

Often families experience loss, anger, denial, anxiety, guilt, grief and depression.[2,36] First, the families lose the patient whom they knew and loved as the patient transforms into a different being when cognitive and functional changes occur. The family experiences grief in losing the individuality of the person as his or her personality changes and his or her memory disappears. Moreover, there is a high degree of depressive symptoms related to the social isolation of caregiving.[74] Finally, there is stress in trying to care for the patient as well as caring for oneself. Sometimes, the stress is from lack of education about the disease. There seems to be a difference in stress levels from spouse caregivers to children caregivers. This may be best accounted for by the fact that adult children feel greater stress perhaps due to multiple demands and responsibilities for caring for their parent family and their own families.[74] Nonetheless, Goy and Ganzini[76] stress the need for ongoing education, as well as reinforcing caregiver training to help reduce the stress.

Albinsson and Strang[77] found that many caregivers have numerous existential concerns. These range from a sense of responsibility, isolation, issues around death and meaning. "Responsibility" included loss of freedom, obligation and guilt, and being faithful to the relationship. "Isolation" included being the only relative, bearing the burden of care, living with a non-communicative being and parenting a parent. "Death issues" included denial of death, trying to live authentically and confronting the patient's preference to die rather than being in a demented state and anticipatory grieving. "Meaning" included the meaning of the illness, routines, memories and passing the person's achievements to others.

Family caregivers may struggle with issues around advance-care planning if the patient's wishes are not clear. Providing clear and realistic information, clarifying patient values to the extent possible, and offering emotional support are essential ways medical professionals can assist families in making difficult decisions.

POTENTIAL RESEARCH ISSUES/OPPORTUNITIES

Ladislaw Volicer, MD and Ann Hurley, RN, PhD, in their seminal work, were leaders in developing innovative and progressive strategies surrounding the end-of-life care of this population. They clearly articulated the difficulty of caring for these patients. Particularly, Volicer and Hurley have articulated four areas challenging the optimal quality of life for these patients. These areas are physical environment, social environment, medical treatment and caregiving. In spite of the dedicated work of Volicer and Hurley, there is a continued understanding that these patients suffer needlessly and that more is needed for education and treatment approaches in these patients.[78]

Given that dementia has not been universally recognized as a terminal disease, research related to optimal end-of-life care for these patients is lacking. However, this is a difficult population to study because these patients constitute a vulnerable population making it difficult to get the approval of investigational review boards. Most of the current research focuses around Alzheimer's dementia; so further studies to evaluate similar issues in the other types of dementia are warranted. Moreover, few prospective studies have been done on this patient population. Most studies have relied on retrospective chart review related to finances, feeding tubes and the use of aggressive hospital care. Medications for slowing the disease are important, particularly for patients with AIDS dementia. However, it would be interesting to determine how much they help in end stage processes. Further research on the use of pain medications for patients with end stage disease would be helpful in defining best practices.

Research into pain and depression has been mostly done within the Advanced Alzheimer's Dementia Unit by Volicer and Hurley.[5] This work has been followed up by pain scale refinement.[51] More research is needed in order to understand and manage other symptoms. It would be important to continue the work of Volicer and Mitchell to develop protocols for feeding with emphasis on critical points of when NOT to insert feeding tubes in patients with advancing dementia. The public lacks knowledge about the benefits and burdens of tube feedings. Research around feeding tubes is particularly important given the public attention to the Schiavo case.

Qualitative studies regarding family decision making about feeding tubes, cardiopulmonary resuscitation, management of recurrent infections would be helpful in guiding other families. Quantitative analysis may also be possible in the areas of caregiver satisfaction, caregiver illness and the use of pain and symptom scales.

Another area of research involves caregivers. The diagnosis of Alzheimer's is in effect a "double death"–the progressive loss of the intactness of the person, and the actual death when the patient is no longer interactive with the world. Studying the family at both points could lead to better understanding of the grief and bereavement process with emphasis on supporting coping strategies. It is also important to evaluate caregiver stress, needs and coping for people from different socioeconomic levels. Further research on the health sequelae of family caregivers could be helpful in determining better support networks. More evaluation of bereavement support for these families could help hospices establish more specific structures.

Finally, since many of these patients are cared for in skilled nursing facilities, it would be helpful to study various clinical pathways to promote best practices in the end stage of various dementias. Many of the quality indicators for long-term care are not appropriate measures or interventions for patients with end stage dementia. Further research on the educational needs of long-term care settings could help nursing adapt other programs such as ELNEC (End of Life Nursing Education Consortium) to better improve the care of dementia patients.

CITED REFERENCES

1. National Institute of Aging and National Institute of Health. *2003 Progress report on Alzheimer's disease.* U.S. Department of Health and Human Services; 2004.

2. Prigerson H. Costs to society of family caregiving for patients with end-stage Alzheimer's disease. *NEJM.* 2003;349(20):1891-1892.

3. American Psychiatric Association. *Diagnostic and Statistical Manual of Mental Disorders.* 4th ed. text revisions. Washington, DC: American Psychiatric Association; 2000.

4. World Health Organization, Regional Office for Southeast Asia. Alzheimer's disease– What is dementia, what is Alzheimer's disease? Mental health and substance abuse. 2005. Available at http://www.Whosea.org/en/section1174/section1199/Section 1167. Accessed January 26, 2006.

5. Volicer L, Hurley A. *Hospice Care for Patients with Advanced Progressive Dementia.* New York, NY: Springer Publishing Company, Inc; 1998.

6. Peterson R. *Mayo Clinics on Alzheimer's disease.* Rochester, Minnesota: Mayo Clinic; 2002.

7. Whalley L, Breitner J. *Dementia.* Oxford, England: Health Press; 2002.

8. Yeaworth R. Dementia: Common types, interventions and advocacy. *Massachusetts Report on Nursing.* 2003;6:18-22.

9. National Institute of Neurological Disorders and Stroke (NINDS). The dementias: Hope through research. Prepared by Office of Communication and Public Liaison, NINDS, NIH. Last updated February 9, 2005. Available at http://www.ninds.nih.gov/disorders/alzheimersdisease. Accessed March 22, 2005.

10. Davies H. Delirium and dementia. In: Stone J, Wyman J, Salisbury S, eds. *Clinical Gerontological Nursing.* Philadelphia, PA: W.B. Saunders; 1999:413-443.

11. Mitchell S, Morris J, Park P, Fries B. Terminal care for persons with advanced dementia in the nursing home and home care settings. *Journal of Palliative Medicine.* 2005;7(6):808-816.

12. Kovach C. Dementia and neurodegenerative illnesses. In: Matzo ML, Sherman DW, eds. *Gerontologic Palliative Care Nursing.* Philadelphia, PA: Mosby Inc; 2004:230-251.

13. Luggen A, Meiner S. Neurological problems. In: Luggen A, Meiner S, eds. *National Geriatric Nursing Association Core Curriculum of Gerontological Nursing.* St. Louis, MO: Mosby; 2001:129–153.

14. Alva G, Potkin S. Alzheimer disease and other dementias. *Clinics in Geriatric Medicine.* 2003;19:763-776.

15. National Institute of Neurological Disorders and Stroke (NINDS). Multi-Infarct Dementia Information Page. Prepared by Office of Communication and Public Liaison, NINDS, NIH. Last updated February 9, 2005. Available at http://www.ninds.nih.gov/disorders/multi_infacrt_dementia. Accessed March 22, 2005.

16. Volicer L, McKee A, Hewitt S. Dementia. *Neurologic Clinics.* 2001;19(4):867-885.

17. Alzheimer's Disease Education and Referral Center *Connections.* 2002;9(4). Available at http://www.alzheimers.org. Accessed May 15, 2005.

18. National Institute of Neurological Disorders and Stroke (NINDS). (2005) Dementia with Lewy Bodies Information Page. Prepared by Office of Communication and Public Liai-

son, NINDS, NIH. Last updated February 9, 2005. Available at http://www.ninds.nih.gov/disorders/dementiawithleweybodies. Accessed March 22, 2005.

19. Luggen A, Miller J, Jett K. General nurse practitioner guidelines: dementia with Lewy bodies. *Geriatric Nursing.* 2004;24(1):56-57.

20. Mendez MF, Cummings JL. *Dementia-A Clinical Approach.* 3rd Ed. Philadelphia, PA: Butterworth-Heinemann; 2003.

21. Sahai-Srivastava S, Jones B. Dementia due to HIV disease. Emedicine. 2004. Available at http://emedicine.com. Accessed March 22, 2005.

22. Forstein M. Psychiatric problems. In: O'Neill J, Selwyn P, Schietinger H, eds. *A Clinical Guide to Supportive and Palliative Care for HIV/AIDS.* Merrifield, VA: Health Resources and Services Administration; 2003:207-252.

23. Folstein M, Folstein S, McHugh PJ. Mini-mental state: A practical method for grading the cognitive state of patients for clinicians. *Journal of Psychiatric Residency.* 1975;12:189-198.

24. National Library of Medicine. Medical Encyclopedia: Dementia. 2004. Available at http://www.nlm.gov./medlineplus/ency. Accessed April 22, 2004

25. Hughes C, Berg L, Danzinger W, Coben L, Martin R. A new clinical scale for staging dementia. *British Journal of Psychiatry.* 1982;140:566-572.

26. Reisberg B, Ferris SH. A clinical scale for symptoms of psychosis in Alzheimer's disease. *Psychopharmacology Bulletin.* 1985;21:101-106.

27. Reisberg B. Functional assessment staging (FAST). *Psychopharmacology Bulletin.* 1988;24:653-659.

28. Luchins D, Hanrahan P. What is the appropriate level of healthcare for end-stage dementia patients? *Journal of the American Geriatric Society.* 1993;41:25-30.

29. Resnick B. Putting research into practice: Behavioral and pharmacological management of dementia. *Geriatric Nursing.* 2004;24(1):58-59.

30. Doody RS, Stevens JC, Beck C, Dubinsky RM, Kaye JA, Gwyther L, et al. Practice parameter: Management of dementia (an evidence-based review). Report of the quality standards subcommittee of the American Academy of Neurology. *Neurology.* 2001;56:1154-1166.

31. Flaskerud JH, Miller EN. Psychosocial and Neuropsychiatric Dysfunction. In: Ungvarski P, Flaskerud J, eds. *HIV/AIDS- A guide to Primary Care Management.* Philadelphia, PA: W.B. Saunders; 1999:255-291.

32. Klein A, Kowell N. Alzheimer's disease and other progressive dementias. In: Volicer L, Hurley A, eds. *Hospice Care for Patients with Advanced Progressive Dementia.* New York, NY: Springer Publishing Company, Inc; 1998:3-28.

33. Moretti R, Torre P, Antonello RM, Cattaruzza T, Cassato G, Bava A. Olanzapine as a possible treatment for anxiety due to vascular dementia: an open study. *American Journal of Alzheimer's Disease and Other Dementias.* 2004;19(20):81-8.

34. DiTrapano D, Guldin A. Treatments for dementia. *New England Advance.* Feb 14, 2005.

35. Finkel S. Behavioral and psychological symptoms of dementia. *Clinics in Geriatric Medicine.* 2003;19:799-824.

36. Volicer L. Management of severe Alzheimer's disease and end-of-life issues. *Clinics in Geriatric Medicine.* 2001;17(2):377-391.

37. Volicer L, Hurley A, Lathi D, Kowall N. Measurement of severity in advanced Alzheimer's disease. *Journal of Gerontology: Medical Sciences.* 2004;49(5):M223-M226.
38. Kovach C, Weissman D, Griffie J, Matson S, Muchka S. Assessment and treatment of discomfort for people with late-stage dementia. *Journal of Pain and Symptom Management.* 1999;18(6),412-419.
39. American Geriatric Society Panel on Persistent Pain in Older Persons. The management of persistent pain in older persons. *Journal of the American Geriatrics Society.* 2002;50(6):S205-S224.
40. Dahlin C. Anxiety, depression and delirium. In: Matzo ML, Sherman DW, eds. *Gerontologic Palliative Care Nursing.* Philadelphia, PA: Mosby Inc; 2004;317-351.
41. Dick K. Dementia. In: Polgar Bailey P, Trybulski J, Sandberg-Cook J, Mahan Buttaro T, eds. *Primary Care: A Collaboration Practice.* Philadelphia, PA: Mosby Inc; 2003:938-942.
42. Sachs G, Shega J, Cox-Hayley D. Barriers to excellent end-of-life care to patients with dementia. *Journal of General Internal Medicine.* 2004:19;1057-1063.
43. Head B. Palliative care for persons with dementia. *Home Healthcare Nurse.* 2003; 21(1):53-60.
44. Smith, S. Providing palliative care for the terminal Alzheimer's patient. In: Volicer L, Hurley A, eds. *Hospice Care for Patients with Advanced Progressive Dementia.* New York, NY: Springer Publishing; 1998:247-256.
45. Mezinkis P, Keller A, Luggen A. Assessment of pain in the cognitively impaired older adult in the long-term care. *Geriatric Nursing.* 2004;25(2):107-112.
46. Graf C, Puntillo K. Pain in the older adult in the intensive care unit. *Critical Care Clinics.* 2003;19:749-770.
47. Evers M, Purohit D, Perl D, Khan K, Martin D. Palliative and aggressive end of life care for patients with dementia. *Psychiatric Services.* 2002;53(5):609-613.
48. Abbey J, Pillar N, DeBellis A, Esterman A, Parker D, Giles Lowcay B. The Abbey Pain Scale - a 1 minute numerical indicator for people with late-stage dementia. *International Journal of Palliative Nursing.* 2004;10(1):6-13.
49. Hurley A, Volicer B, Hanrahan P, Houde S, Volicer L. Assessment of discomfort in advanced Alzheimer patients. *Research in Nursing and Health.* 2004;15(5):369-377.
50. Feldt K. The checklist of nonverbal pain indicators (CNPI). *Pain Management Nursing.* 2000;1(1):13-21.
51. Warden V, Hurley A, Volcier L. Development and psychometric evaluation of the pain assessment in advanced dementia (PAINAD) scale. *Journal of the American Medical Directors Association.* 2003;4(1):9-15.
52. Lane P, Kuntupis M, MacDonald S, McCarthy P, Panke J, Warden V, Volicer L. A pain assessment tool for people with advanced Alzheimer's and other progressive dementias. *Home Healthcare Nurse.* 2003;1(21):32-37.
53. Hurley A, Volicer L. Alzheimer Disease-"It's okay, mama, if you want to go, it's okay." *JAMA.* 2002;288(18):2324-2331.
54. Lentz J. Daily baths: torment or comfort at the end of life? *Journal of Hospice and Palliative Nursing.* 2002;5(1):34-39.

55. Twillman R, Long T, Cathers T, Meuller D. Treatment of painful skin ulcers with topical opioids. *Journal of Pain and Symptom Management.* 1999;17(4):288-292.

56. Costa PT Jr, Williams TF, Somerfield M, et al. *Early Identification of Alzheimer's Disease and Related Dementias. Clinical Practice Guideline No. 19.* Rockville, MD: Department of Health and Human Services, Public Health Agency, Agency for Health Care Policy and Research. AHCPR Publication No. 97-0703. 1996.

57. Pinderhughes S, Morrison S. Evidence-based approach to management of fever in patients with end-stage dementia. *Journal of Palliative Medicine.* 2003;6(3):351-354.

58. Morrison S, Sui A. Survival in end-stage dementia following acute illness. *JAMA.* 2000;284(1):47-52.

59. Van der Steen J, Ooms M, van der Wal G, Ribbe M. Pneumonia: the demented patient's best friend? Discomfort after starting or withdrawing antibiotic treatment. *Journal of the American Geriatric Society.* 2002;50:1681-1688.

60. Lacey D. Tube feeding, antibiotics, and hospitalization of nursing home residents with end-stage dementia: perceptions of key medical decision-makers. *American Journal of Alzheimer's Disease and other Dementias.* 2005;20(4):211-219.

61. Ahronheim J, Morrison S, Baskin S, Morris J, Meier D. Treatment of the dying in the acute care hospital: advanced dementia. *Archives of Internal Medicine.* 1996;156(18):2094-2100.

62. Johnson S. Making room for dying: end of life care in nursing homes. Improving end of life care: why it has been so difficult? *Hastings Center Report Special Report.* 2005;35(6):S37-S41.

63. Gillick, M. Sounding board. Rethinking the role of tube feeding in patients with advanced dementia. *NEJM.* 2000;342(3):206-210.

64. Campbell M, Guzman J. A proactive approach to improve end-of-life care in a medical intensive care unit for patients with terminal dementia. *Critical Care Medicine.* 2004;32(9):1839-1843.

65. Brotons M, Kroger S. The impact of music therapy on language functioning in dementia. *The Journal of Music Therapy.* 2000;37(3):183-195.

66. Kirkland K, McIiveen. Full circle: spiritual therapy for people with dementia. *American Journal of Alzheimer's Disease.* 1999;14:245-247.

67. Kolanowski A, Litaker M, Buettner L. Efficacy of theory-based activities for behavioral symptoms of dementia. *Nursing Research.* 2005;54(4):219-228.

68. Schulz R, Mendelsohn A, Haley W, Mahoney D, Allen R, Zhang S, Thompson L, Belle S. End of life care and effects of bereavement on family caregiver of persons with dementia. *NEJM.* 2003; 349:1936-1942.

69. National Hospice Organization. *Medical Guidelines for Determining Prognosis in Selected Non-Cancer Diseases.* Arlington, Virginia: National Hospice Organization; 1996:12-13.

70. Berkelman D, Black B, Shore A, Kasper J, Rabins P. Hospice care in a cohort of elders with dementia and mild cognitive impairment. *Journal of Pain and Symptom Management.* 2005;30(3):208-213.

71. Volicer L, Hurley A, Zuzka B. End-of-life care for patients with advanced dementia. *JAMA.* 2000;284(19):2449-2450.

72. Hanrahan P, Raymond M, McGowan Luchins D. Criteria for enrolling dementia patients in hospice: a replication. *American Journal of Hospice and Palliative Care.* 1999;16(1):395-400.

73. National Hospice and Palliative Care Organization. *Newsline.* 2004;15(7);1.

74. Diwan S, Hougham G, Sachs G. Strain experienced by caregivers of dementia patients receiving palliative care: findings from the palliative excellence in Alzheimer care efforts (PEACE) program. *Journal of Palliative Medicine.* 2005;7(6):797-807.

75. Heyman A, Peterson B, Fillenbaum G. Pieper C. Predictors of time to institutionalization of patients with Alzheimer's disease: the CERAD experience, part XVII. *Neurology.* 1997;48:527-532.

76. Goy E, Ganzini L. End-of-life care in geriatric psychiatry. *Clinics in Geriatric Medicine.* 2003;19:841-856.

77. Albinsson L, Strang P. Existential concerns of families of late-stage dementia patients: Questions of freedom, choices, isolation, death, and meaning. *Journal of Palliative Medicine.* 2003;6(2):225-235.

78. Aminoff BZ, Adunsky A. Dying dementia patients: too much suffering, too little palliation. *American Journal of Alzheimer's Disease and other Dementias.* 2004;19(4):243-7.